Contents

Naturally Straight Hair

Discover a Revolutionary New Way to Press Your Hair Without the Use of Heat

DeShond C. Barnes

Lulu.com

Published by Lulu.com

ISBN: 978-0-557-32617-4

Introduction

Many people press their hair on a regular basis, but the fact is – most people who press their hair don't like the intense heat exposure that goes along with it as heat exposure can cause severe damage to the hair. Most people who press their hair could never imagine a way of getting the benefits of pressed hair without the heat exposure. But what if that were possible? What if you could press your hair in a way that does not involve the use of heat? Well you are about to learn how to do just that!

Hi. My name is DeShond C. Barnes. I am an African-American male who presses his hair, however, I use no pressing comb, no blow dryer, no heat of any kind. All I use is a special shampoo, hair oil and a natural comb. I combine the special shampoo, hair oil and special hair combing techniques that leave my hair so *ultra-silky* soft and smooth that it looks and feels as though it has been *pressed with a pressing comb!* My hair is left so ultra-silky soft and smooth that if I shake my head, I can feel my hair *vibrating*. This revolutionary new method of pressing your hair will plunge your hair in ultra-silky softness and smoothness, and will eliminate the need for blow dryers and pressing combs – thus eliminating the potential for hair damage.

Whenever I visit my stylist for a haircut, I have to be careful not to get my hair too straight – or he/she won't be able to cut it! Time and time again, stylists have asked me the following questions: "Have you ever had a perm?" and "Do you use anything else in your hair besides oil?" I simply answer "no" to the questions. If this revolutionary new hair pressing method has the effect that it has on *my* hair (and I'm a *male*) – just imagine the effect that it would have on *females'* hair!

Aren't you just itching to learn more about this hair pressing method? Well now I will provide you with complete details about it! I will explain it to you by breaking it down into a series of *steps*. First, you will need the following items: (1) *Alberto VO5 Herbal escapes free me freesia Moisturizing shampoo* (15 fl oz.), *Pro-Line Hair Food* (Nutrition Capillaire – 4.5 oz.), an extra large hand mirror (the type of hand mirror that is used in barber and beauty salons – available at major beauty supply stores) and a *FirstLine evolve Essentials Detangling and Dresser Comb* (2 pack).

If you are a resident of the United States, then you can find *Alberto VO5 Herbal escapes free me freesia Moisturizing shampoo* in the *non-ethnic* hair products section at *Ultra Foods, Albertsons* grocery stores, *CVS Pharmacy, Kmart* and other local retail stores. If you are a resident of the United Kingdom, then you can purchase *Alberto VO5 Herbal escapes free me freesia Moisturizing shampoo* from www.Amazon.co.uk. Simply type "free me freesia shampoo" in the home page search field and press "Enter." *Alberto VO5 Herbal escapes free me freesia Moisturizing shampoo* contains extracts from *freesia* and other flowers and leaves. Shampoos that contain extracts from flowers and leaves tend to give your hair the ability to be "naturally" pressed. *Alberto VO5 Herbal escapes free me freesia Moisturizing shampoo* also contains an ingredient called *biotin*, which – according to research studies - helps to prevent your hair from turning gray!

If you are a resident of the United States, then you can find *Pro-Line Hair Food* in the *ethnic* hair products section of *numerous* local retail stores and beauty supply stores (this product has a *very* high distribution). If you are a resident of the United Kingdom, then you can purchase *Pro-Line Hair Food* from www.Amazon.co.uk. *Pro-Line Hair Food* contains *flammable* ingredients. Oils that leave your hair *flammable* tend to give your hair the ability to be "naturally" pressed.

If you are a resident of the United States, then you can find a *FirstLine evolve Essentials Detangling and Dresser Comb* (2 pack) at some *Walmart* stores. If you are a resident of the United Kingdom, then look for a *FirstLine evolve Essentials Detangling and Dresser Comb* at your local UK *Walmart* store. If it is not there, then you can purchase it at www.PakCosmetics.com. This comb comes in packs of two. They are both purple colored. One of them has a *handle*… while the other does not. The one that has the *handle* is the one to use for your hair. The UPC (Universal Product Code) for *Alberto VO5 Herbal escapes free me freesia Moisturizing shampoo* is: 022400340067. The UPC for

Pro-Line Hair Food is: 072982000323. The UPC for the *FirstLine evolve Essentials Detangling and Dresser Comb* (2 pack) is: 761809045295 (product number 529).

Step 1

Rinse hair thoroughly with warm water from your kitchen sink (allow water to *continue* to *run* after your hair has been thoroughly rinsed). *Fill* one of your palms with a *generous* amount of *Alberto VO5 Herbal escapes free me freesia Moisturizing shampoo,* then rub both palms together. Stick your head *back* under the running water for 5 more seconds (without *touching* your hair), then remove your head from the running water stream and massage the shampoo (that you have *already* applied to *both* hands) into your hair and scalp – working the shampoo into a lather. Lather for 8 seconds, then rinse hair thoroughly with warm water. Continue massaging your hair and scalp while rinsing.

After rinsing hair thoroughly, *repeat* the entire process outlined in the *previous* paragraph (water should *continue* to run)… but this time you will use a *much smaller quantity* of shampoo than you did the *first* time. This time, you will only use the amount of shampoo equivalent to the size of a *quarter*. Repeat the process one final time… using the amount of shampoo equivalent to the size of a *penny* this time. You will notice that as you repeat the process, your shampoo lathers become *richer* each time (with *less* shampoo each time). After lathering and rinsing a total of 3 times, *press down* on your hair (using both hands) for 2 seconds to remove the *excess* water from your hair, then *lightly* towel-dry for about 15 seconds. Your hair should be left *slightly moist*, instead of *completely dry*. Leaving your hair *slightly* moist after washing makes it easier to "naturally" press your hair.

Step 2

Apply a *generous* amount of *Pro-Line Hair Food* to one of your palms, then rub both palms together and massage into hair and scalp. Massage for 3 minutes. Wash hands.

Step 3

Remove the shade covering your *bathroom* lights (if possible). This will give you extra brightness so that you can see your hair better (the *bathroom* usually provides better lighting than any other room in the house or apartment). Grab an extra large hand mirror, then stand in front of your bathroom cabinet's mirror (looking directly into the mirror). Turn to one side, hold the hand mirror in front of your face, then turn the hand mirror slightly to one side so that you can see the complete side of your head in the bathroom cabinet mirror. Using a *FirstLine evolve Essentials Detangling and Dresser Comb* (the one with the *handle*) begin combing the top, side and back of your hair on *that* side of your head – combing it all towards the *back* using one side of the comb (you will be holding the hand mirror up with one hand, and combing your hair with the other).

After several strokes, turn your body around so that you can see the *other* side of your head in the bathroom cabinet mirror. Begin combing the top, side and back of your hair on *that* side of your head – combing it all towards the *back* using the *other* side of the comb.

After several strokes, turn your body back around so that you can see the *first*-combed side of your head again. Begin combing the top, side and back of your hair on *that* side of your head – combing it all towards the *back* using the *original* side of the comb, but this time you will gradually work your way over to the *other* side of your head (using the *same* side of the comb), then gradually work your way back over to the original side of your head. Turn your body back around so that you can see the *second*-combed side of your head again, then do the same

thing for *that* side using the *second-*
used side of the comb.

Step 4

Now turn your body back around so that you can see the *first*-combed side of your head again. Begin combing the top, side and back of your hair on *that* side of your head – but this time you will comb it all towards the *front* using the *original* side of the comb. Turn your body back around so that you can see the *second*-combed side of your head again, then do the same thing for *that* side using the *second*-used side of the comb.

Turn your body back around so that you can see the *first*-combed side of your head again. Begin combing the top, side and back of your hair on *that* side of your head – combing it all towards the *front* using the *original* side of the comb, but this time you will gradually work your way over to the *other* side of your head (using the *same* side of the comb), then gradually work your way back over to the original side of your head.

Turn your body back around so that you can see the *second*-combed side of your head again, then do the same thing for *that* side using the *second*-used side of the comb. Now turn your body back around so that you can see the *first*-combed side of your head again, then comb it all towards the *back* again (repeat step 3).

Step 5

Reapply a generous amount of *Pro-Line Hair Food* to one of your palms, then rub both palms together and massage into hair and scalp. Massage for 3 minutes. Wash hands. You can use *slightly* less *Pro-Line Hair Food* this time than you did the *first* time.

Wipe the oil residue from the top of your comb using a piece of tissue paper, then rinse the oil residue from the other parts of your comb using warm water. Be sure to rinse both sides of the comb, then thoroughly dry the comb with a towel and repeat steps 3 and 4. It is very important that you not rinse your comb until *after* you have *r*eapplied *Pro-Line Hair Food* to your hair, massaged it in and washed your hands.

Step 6

Wipe the oil from your forehead using a moist towel, then turn your body around so that you can see the *first*-combed side of your head again. Begin combing from the *middle* of the top of your head *over* towards *that* side, and from the *middle* of the back of your head *over* towards *that* side (using one side of the comb). After several strokes, begin combing from *that* side back over towards the *middle* of the *top* of your head, and from *that* side back over towards the *middle* of the back of your head (using that *same* side of the comb).

Now – using the *other* side of the comb – begin combing from the middle of the top of your head *over* towards *that* side again, and from the middle of the back of your head *over* towards *that* side again. After several strokes, begin combing from *that* side back over towards the middle of the top of your head, and from *that* side back over towards the middle of the back of your head (using that *same* side of the comb).

Step 7

Turn your body around so that you can see the *second*-combed side of your head again, then apply step 6 to *that* side of your head. Now turn your body back around so that you can see the *first*-combed side of your head again, then comb it all towards the back again (repeat step 3).

Now your hair is ready for that special style you're seeking! You will notice that steps 6 and 7 will release the pressed *look* and *feel* to your hair. Combing your hair in directions that go *against* its natural growth pattern adds *bulk* and *straightness* to your hair, especially when you comb from the middle of your head *over* towards the sides (and visa versa), using *both* sides of the comb. But you must comb in *all* of the directions (only after shampooing) to get the full effect! When you combine those hair combing techniques with the extracts from flowers and leaves that are found in *Alberto VO5 Herbal escapes free me freesia Moisturizing shampoo,* and the *flammable* ingredients that are found in *Pro-Line Hair Food,* the end result is hair that is so *ultra*-silky soft and smooth that it looks and feels as though it has been pressed with a pressing comb!

Daily Maintenance

To maintain your hair's pressed look and feel, repeat steps 2, 3 and 4 daily. Steps 6 and 7 (combing over towards the sides and visa versa) should be done *only* after shampooing. So, if you shampoo your hair once per week (as I do), you should follow *all* steps (1 through 7) *once* per week – *only* on the day that you shampoo. On all other days, it is only necessary to follow steps 2, 3 and 4. It is *very* important that you not shampoo *daily*. Daily shampooing is *extremely* harsh on your hair and can *strip* your hair of its natural moisture (especially if you have *ethnic* hair).

Also, it is very important that you *briefly* comb through your hair right before shampooing. This will *stir up the oils* that you *already* applied to your hair *earlier* in that day. Stirring up the oils in your hair right before shampooing tends to leave your hair softer and more manageable after shampooing, thus allowing for *optimum* "natural" pressing results! When you briefly comb through your hair right before shampooing, you only have to comb it towards the back, then towards the front, then back towards the back again for a total of about 8 minutes or so (using *both* sides of the comb). Your only purpose of doing that is to stir up the oils right before shampooing, but you have to have *already* applied *Pro-Line Hair Food* to your hair earlier in that day. So try to shampoo your hair in the *afternoons* or *evenings*, instead of in the *mornings*.

Also, be sure that it is not *hot* and/or *humid* inside of your house or apartment on the day that you shampoo. Heat and humidity will make it harder to achieve optimum results. If the weather is hot and/or humid on the day that you shampoo, make sure that you use *air conditioning* after shampooing (while combing your hair) to achieve *optimum* results! Whenever you are outside on days when the weather is hot and/or humid… and your hair *reverts* as a result, all you have to do to return your hair to its original state is to stir up the oils (as explained previously). You do *not* have to *reapply* oil to your hair, instead, just stir up the oils that you *already* applied to your hair *earlier* that day.

Also, try as much as possible to minimize your hair's physical contact with *precipitation* (especially *rain*). Try using a *bubble* umbrella, instead of a traditional *nylon* umbrella. Bubble umbrellas offer *more* protection for your hair than nylon umbrellas because bubble umbrellas *come all the way down around you*, making it very difficult for *wind-driven* precipitation to make physical contact with your hair! Bubble umbrellas are available at a variety of retail stores in the United States, including *Walmart* and *Target*. If you are a resident of the United Kingdom, and you are unable to find them at your local retail stores, you can purchase them at www.Amazon.co.uk. Simply search under "bubble umbrella."

Another way to maintain your hair's pressed look and feel is to wear your hair going towards the *back* a few days per week (every other day – if you like). In other words, try not to wear your hair in the *exact same direction* each day. It is necessary to apply a *generous* amount of *Pro-Line Hair Food* to your hair *only* after shampooing. On all other days, you can apply a *smaller* amount of *Pro-Line Hair Food* to your hair.

If you have any questions or comments, please e-mail them to me at nathanael.eh.123@gmail.com. Please put "about your book" in the subject line. **I would love to hear from you!**

GOOD LUCK WITH YOUR HAIR!!!